Lebowitz, Sally E.

Friend of the family

FRIEND of the FAMILY

A Hospice Volunteer's Experience

SALLY E. LEBOWITZ

Written by
MARY-ALICE HERBERT

LAUREL PRESS, INC.
Bethel Park, Pennsylvania

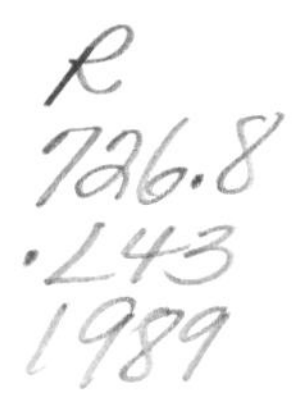

Cover illustration by Mary Scurlock

Cover design by Ed Macko

Book design by Pat Polito and Chuck McAdams

Published by Laurel Press, Inc., 1514 Holly Hill Drive, Bethel Park, PA 15102.

FIRST EDITION

Library of Congress Cataloging-in-Publication Data
Lebowitz, Sally E.
Friend of the Family: A Hospice Volunteer's Experience / Sally E. Lebowitz. 1st ed.

Bibliography.

Includes index.

1. Hospice care—United States.
2. Social work with the terminally ill—United States.
3. Home care services—United States.

I. Title.
R726.8.L43 1989 362.1'75—dc20 89-8173

ISBN 0-9619155-1-X

Printed and bound in the United States of America.

To Martin and Barbara

and

To the patients, families, and volunteers
whose love and work continue to be an inspiration.

CONTENTS

Writer's Preface vix

Acknowledgments vii

Contents vi

Prologue 3
The hospice concept...

CHAPTER 1 Ann Banks 9
A good beginning.

CHAPTER 2 Friends 17
Who becomes a hospice volunteer?

CHAPTER 3 Virginia Fremont 29
A cultivated lady.

CHAPTER 4 Gifts 35
What can a volunteer do?

CHAPTER 5 Emma Gruber 47
A woman of spirit.

CHAPTER 6 Rewards 53
Why is hospice work so gratifying?

CHAPTER 7 Arthur Wilcox 63
An unhappy experience.

CHAPTER 8 Perspectives 69
How does a volunteer handle stress?

CHAPTER 9 Mr. Miller 81
A family man.

CHAPTER 10 Choices 87
When is hospice the right way?

Epilogue 97
...peace of mind.

Resources 101

Index 105

ACKNOWLEDGMENTS

Countless personal and professional friends helped to bring this book to completion. To these are owed a particular debt:

Lynn Abram at the South Hills Family Hospice; Ira Bates at the National Hospice Organization; Bill Halamandaris at the Foundation for Hospice and Homecare; Robert Hilberg, M.D.; Ann Katterhagen, at Memorial Medical Center of Springfield, Illinois; Della Mussitch; Carol Pasinski; Rabbi William Sajowitz; Elaine Supowitz, Professor of English; Joan L. Williamson; Connie Yarbro, Editor of *Seminars in Oncology Nursing.*

The greatest contributions to this book must go unacknowledged by name—to them is owed deepest gratitude.

WRITER'S PREFACE

FRIEND OF THE FAMILY is **about** *people of great courage, people who, knowing they are dying of cancer, want a good death—one filled with life, with family, and with friends. It is also written for them and for those like them who respect the courage of that choice and want to help, yet perhaps hesitate because the subject seems too sensitive to approach.*

For those from many walks of life who are hospice volunteers, or who would be hospice volunteers if they had foundation enough to decide, this book shares experience and insights.

For those in the health professions, the social services, education, and the clergy who would like to help dying patients' families decide among alternative kinds of care, this book offers insight into what it is like to be cared for and to die in one's own home and, too, what it is like, with the help of professionals and volunteers, to provide that care at home.

And, for those who are free to choose—although they may feel as if they have no choices left—this book offers a chance to consider the personal aspects of choosing between dying in a hospital and dying at home.

This account of Sally's experience is authentic. It represents truthfully her challenges, her emotions, her personality. She is a real, not an ideal, volunteer. And no two volunters are alike. Her strengths and her weaknesses—she freely admits both—are her own. Her style is her own. She alone, and no organization for which she has worked, is responsible for her point of view. Factual details have been altered, and meticulously so, to guard the privacy and dignity of Sally's friends, both living and dead. The stories of her patients are composites—collages, not photographs—and in no way identify actual persons. What is at once personal and universal, however, is the courage of patients and their families to meet the final time of life as a challenge—daring to seek comfort, meaning and peace.

MARY-ALICE HERBERT
April 1989

FRIEND of the FAMILY

A Hospice Volunteer's Experience

PROLOGUE

LIFE ENDS. Whatever our faith, whatever our system of belief, life as we know it ends. People enter life, and they leave it. Accepting that, respecting that, is central to the work of hospice. The work itself, however, is concerned with life, with what is, rather than what is not. It is concerned with the life of the dying person, a life that goes on until it goes on no more. It is concerned with the lives it touches, lives of family and friends—lives that continue to go on.

Hospice begins when nothing more *of a curative nature* can be done to change the course of a disease, usually cancer, and when there is certainty, or near certainty, of death. There is, however, much more *of a human nature* that can be done—and what is done will help to give that death, like life, its own special shape and color. Such a death need not be lonely, mechanistic, miserable: it can be dignified, peaceful, even noble. Death, like all the other passages of our lives, is a challenge to our humanity. We can better it with work, with imagination, and with care.

Hospice means comfort and care for the dying and the family of the dying. The medieval word *hospes,* which meant a shelter, a temporary home for travelers, bears the seed of our word *hospital,* a word we associate with treatment—and often with pain, fear, and loss of hope. From *hospes* also came *hospitality,* the idea of an open door, a warm hearth, a place of comfort, rest and care—and of people, warm of heart, open of mind, generous of spirit. That, too, is temporary, ending with the traveler's leave-taking. It is significant, however, that the early word *hospes* also meant, both *guest* and *host,* as if the role each played in meeting was to exchange something of mutual importance. Less significant was the separateness of their roles—the one to travel on and the other to remain behind to shelter other travelers.

Today, hospice means more home-like than hospital-like care. And hospice is a concept more than a place. Hospice programs can be found in facilities specially built to provide home-like care, and in hospitals with specially dedicated wings. Hospice can also be found in patients' own homes. The concept always includes the element of home, but that can occur anywhere family and friends, supportive professionals and volunteers meet at the bedside of the dying patient for the exchange of comfort and care. Those who provide care usually include family members (although not necessarily) and almost always volunteers and nurses. Often there is a social worker; sometimes a counselor, therapist, or member of the clergy.

For eight years I have worked under a hospice program run by a hospital for people who have chosen to die in their own homes. Our program began by helping only patients with cancer; today we have added patients with AIDS. Family, nurses, social workers, volunteers—whoever is involved function as a team, under the guidance of a medical director and the attending physician. Volunteers have access to a coordinator, who also initially provides for training, and staff who advise and guide as the case progresses. Our concern—the shared concern of the team—is the *quality of life* for that patient, both physical and emotional. Our focus is always relieving pain and providing comfort. We stand by the patient, the family and one another.

This book is meant to provide the kind of personal account that is needed among the many other kinds of information available about hospice and the materials used for the training of volunteers and professionals who work with dying patients. As the story unfolds, I hope my readers will feel included in an experience, having been along on a journey of discovery, meeting beautiful, sad, funny people, learning dozens of tiny truths, and a few great ones. Although it is completely my story—the experiences of two volunteers even within the same program can never be the same—so much of the experience is, at heart, universal. I want to provide my readers with that sense of having been there.

This is my story.

Chapter 1

Ann Banks

1

ANN BANKS

I SPENT TWO WEEKS in intensive training as a volunteer, half-day sessions that left me exhausted. I knew I was learning more than I ever had—about cancer, and life, and people, and myself. Before I expected it, I got the call for my first case ....

I drove slowly down the street counting houses. One ... two ... three ... to the fourth one on the left. I pulled up beside a small, neat brick Cape Cod with a carefully trimmed lawn. I turned my wheels against the downhill slope. I set the emergency brake against possible drifting. I tightened the windows against the possibility of rain. I started digging for a comb, and I stopped myself. *Go, just go.* I took the flagstone steps (seventeen of them) deliberately. *I wish I had one more day to prepare myself. How can I possibly help someone to die!*

Then the door was open. There stood a slim young woman, dressed in faded jeans and a man's white, dress shirt. She had soft, brown eyes and a gentle smile, and as she held her arms open to me, she said, "I just know you're the lady from hospice. I'm so glad you're here. I'm Ann."

It was perfectly natural for us to hold one another and to cry a little. My tension washed away.

I remember very little specifically about that first visit. I don't believe I said very much—but I felt the grace of knowing the right words when there was something I could say. And, I felt like a friend who shows up at just the right moment.

As I returned to the car, I felt quiet and competent. I had taken the first step and I knew I would somehow take the rest. I seldom doubted again that in choosing hospice work I had chosen to do the right thing.

I visited three times, a week apart, before Ann's husband died. Ed was in no pain. He slept and slept, only occasionally aware of what was happening around him.

Ann cared for him gently. She was half his age and half his height, yet she touched him and moved him with firm, deliberate hands. She was light and graceful on her feet, and she smiled softly, and often. She was in perfect control. She treated me like a guest, making coffee and nutbread for my visits. At first I didn't really feel needed. Ann almost seemed to be entertaining me. In her low, rich voice, she told me all the best about her life with Ed—her meeting and marrying him, the delight they shared in their son, their vacations to the shore, their local jaunts on weekends—the happy moments of a family of three.

On my third visit, Ed was resting quietly as usual, his room freshly aired and the scent of fabric softener still on the sheets. It was Good Friday, so their son Billy was home from school. Billy, at 9, was a quiet, independent little person, content to read by himself in the den. To Ann, however, Ed appeared "fitful" and Billy "restless." To me, Ann seemed the uneasy one—she was out of coffee, and there was no fresh bread.

I recognized an opportunity to do some active helping. I convinced Ann to sit with Ed while I took Billy to do the shopping and one or two other errands.

"I'm glad you brought me," he said. "I've been waiting to get my mom flowers for Easter. But she's always with me and there's no one to take me."

Billy told me about some neighbors who used to visit regularly.

"They used to tell me to help my mom. But anyway, my mom does everything. She doesn't really need any help. But she cries sometimes. I know it because her eyes get real red."

I was very happy to do something for that child. I began to realize what I was doing for his mother just by coming, and listening, and sharing her delicious breads. Still, helping, to me, has always meant the roll-up-the-sleeves-and-dig-in variety.

Billy chose a pot of bright yellow chrysanthemums. We went to McDonald's for burgers and fries and Coke, just in time to spoil our dinners. When Billy scampered up the long stone climb with his pot of flowers at a precarious angle, he called over his shoulder, "Now my mom will cry because she's happy!"

Ed died quietly in his sleep that night.

He had planned every detail of his life, including the days following his death. He had arranged for his own final business to transpire automatically; a single phone call to his lawyer activated insurance companies, banks, and the mortuary. He left nothing for Ann to do. She was free to go on with her life.

Ann was sad, very sad to lose Ed. But she was as well-prepared as anyone could hope to be. She had done what she could for him. In retrospect, I realize Ann's uneasiness the last time I was there may have come from a sense, on some level, that Ed was about to die. She may have wanted to be alone to say good-bye.

I have never forgotten the lessons of that first case. Just by being there and listening, by putting myself at another's disposal, without plans of my own, to do whatever there is to do, or to do nothing at all—this is helping. Others may stop visiting out of fear and helplessness, and, really, who can blame them? But that special friend of the family, the hospice volunteer, is there. And you can count on that.

Chapter 2

Friends

2

FRIENDS

IN TODAY'S SOCIETY, where anything worth doing is worth doing for money, volunteer work is something of an enigma. In a society in which *death* and *cancer* are almost unspeakable words, that volunteers choose work with terminally ill cancer patients is even more puzzling. People ask, "Why do you do it?"

When I lived in Connecticut in 1965, I read about hospice in England. That was before hospice came to this country. It was the concept that attracted me. Dying at home, with family support and professional care—and caring friends.

Reading about it and thinking about it, I said, "I'm going to become involved—some way—in that wonderful work." At the time I had two little babies and our life was very unsettled ... there was no way I could get involved in anything more. But I knew one day I would.

My life, too, has been touched personally by cancer. I have a very dear friend who has had cancer for 28 years. She has held the disease at bay and kept it a secret because of the threat it could mean to her professional career. It is very difficult for her. As her checkups approach every three months, her fear and apprehension build. I learned about hospice for her, partly, and I also learned about cancer for her. Hospice training is largely learning about cancer.

Some twelve or fifteen years after I first heard of hospice, I was living here in Pennsylvania and I became involved in the early planning of a hospice near my home. I was enthusiastic about the concept. I didn't know then about lay volunteers. I wanted to do something directly, though, and I was frustrated. I wasn't a doctor, a nurse, a social worker, or a member of the clergy. I felt unsure that I could make a real contribution.

I was a dental hygienist. One of my patients, a doctor (and a heavy smoker) told me something that strengthened my resolve—although at the time it made me want to choke him. He said that he was relieved to know that volunteers were available to visit cancer patients because he personally could not stand to be around people dying from cancer.

"When they get to a certain point," he said, "I put them in the hospital and never see them again."

When he told me that, I think the color must have drained from my face and I had to leave the room. I told the girls at the front desk never to put him in my chair again.

That's when I knew I had to volunteer. I knew there was an enormous need for those who could help to do so. Not everyone could help. I knew I could help, therefore, I felt I must. That is why I still do it—because I *can.*

Although I did not know anyone connected with hospice when I heard about it and wanted to become involved, many people who volunteer have had family members die of cancer. Many of those, in fact, have experienced hospice in their own families. Volunteers are often surviving spouses and children who are grateful that hospice was there for them. They want to give something back, they need to, and they know they can. If their own lives had not been touched, they may have never become involved. They may never have known how greatly volunteers were—and are—needed.

Wanting to give, to nurture, needing to be important, to make a difference, to be special—all these are expressed by people who learn they can offer something, and therefore, they feel they must. Being in touch with their own needs, they respond to the needs of others—to the benefit of both.

But the response to the very idea on the part of people whose lives have not been touched is often shock, a mixture of fear and horror, "I could never do what you do."

The hospice volunteer hears those words again and

again. "It must take a very special person," they say. They think, *not me.*

Yet those who volunteer do not consider themselves extraordinary. Not everyone can do this kind of work, to be sure. To that extent it takes a special person. But more people need to know that it's such an important kind of work. It needs to be talked about and understood. More people need to know that this work is positive—it is not morbid or depressing. Yes, it is very sad to see people sick and alone. But we can change that loneliness with companionship and comfort. Yes, it is sad to see a family in stress, but we can change that, too, by giving them relief.

And those who volunteer are seldom without some hesitation. Death is mystifying, and the unknown is truly frightening. The key to it, I think, is being able to face your own mortality—and you might need help to do that. This is what part of my training was all about. In one of the sessions, for instance, we had to write our own obituaries. That disturbed some trainees. I remember someone who just walked out and never came back. For me it wasn't too hard, but it took some people a while to get used to the idea.

Otherwise, the volunteers that I know are just ordinary, well-rounded people. They do a lot of different things. Most of these are not people whose whole lives are dedicated to helping people although a few are. I know that I can't give everything to hospice work. I have a small business, a large family, and many friends—hospice is one of the things I do. I do it because I love to do it. I have time for it because I make time for it. It is not my life, but it is an important part of my life.

Who are some of the others?

Most, although definitely not all, are women. Often, although certainly not always, they are mothers of grown or almost grown children.

* A friend, Kathy, mother of two and nurse employed full time in the coronary care unit in a local hospital, is a hospice volunteer. Volunteer nurses are an especially caring and willing group of volunteers.

* Della, another friend, who is not employed outside her home, is a wife, a mother of three, a volunteer Christian education teacher, and a very respected hospice volunteer.

* Another woman, married and without children, an amateur golf champion, volunteers extensively, in both a hospital and a home-based hospice program.

Some of the male volunteers are retired men whose wives died on the hospice program. A few are businessmen who volunteer evenings and weekends.

* One man, a mill-worker, and a quiet and gentle man, devastated by his wife's death, so respected and loved the

volunteer who served in that family that he too is a volunteer and dedicated to being as good.

* Another man, a sharp, successful businessman who also lost his wife, has become a sensitive and caring volunteer.

* Don, a single retired businessman who loves baking, gardening, and playing cards, has made a family of his hospice patients.

Clearly, there is no "typical" volunteer. Lynn Abram, now a friend, who as hospice volunteer coordinator of the South Hills Family Hospice guided me through training and many cases, says this about volunteers:

"The typical volunteer is anyone and everyone. From 21 to 100 years old. With a master's degree, or without a high school diploma. Man or woman. Black or white. Catholic, Jew, or Protestant—from Christian Scientist to Born Again Christian—or without any particular religious belief at all." So much for demographics.

But volunteers are special. Maybe not extraordinary, but indeed special. Circumstance, if not destiny, selects people and challenges them to become exceptions. People who have once been helped, who might not otherwise have thought of volunteering, want to help in return. Nurses, whose busy routine daytime jobs sometimes frustrate them, are drawn after hours to bedsides where there is time to take time—time to talk and to listen. Mothers who have finely developed nurturing qualities want to continue giving—and giving, perhaps, where it is really appreciated, not taken for granted. Men who have met the traditional demands upon their time may find time after that job is done to develop another "softer" side.

To be a *good* volunteer, however, requires that a person be, first and foremost, "a good, basic human being." Someone responsible and dependable, someone to count on. Lynn explains, "I don't have very much patience with people who don't get there when they're supposed to. If they can't do that, they can't do anything!"

In addition, there are special characteristics that she looks for in a potential volunteer.

- Availability. To have or to be able to make the time.
- Flexibility. To be comfortable with a variety of people and settings.
- An accepting, non-judgmental attitude.
- Ability to communicate well—especially to listen.
- Warmth.
- Compassion for people and their problems.
- Willingness to help people in pain.
- Ability to serve on a team. (You can't want to keep patients to yourself.)
- A sense of humor.

It is the sense of humor that may come as a surprise.

Working with pain and stress would be intolerable for me without it. You have to be able to laugh. You have to be able to shift gears and laugh. My friend Barbara, who is a full-time volunteer with a large case load and who does wonderful work, said, "You must tell them in the book how we love to get together and tell jokes—and eat hot fudge sundaes!" So I am.

Some people are not suited for hospice work. Those who know that, of course, don't become involved. Some have misconceptions about the role of the volunteer, however. Screening by trained professionals is needed if a program is to detect those misconceptions and determine whether an applicant for volunteer work is suitable for training. Screening is the first important stage of a solid program. It goes a long way to protect everyone involved.

When I was screened, for instance, I was asked about deaths in my family. When I talked about my father's death four years before, I came across as having worked through the grief process successfully. People who are motivated to volunteer because of having had someone die in the family may first need time to do their own grief work. The purpose of volunteer work is to help others, not to get over someone's death. You have to take care of that first, then, having grown through that experience, give of yourself.

Training, too, helps to select out those who are not suited—or not yet ready. Because of the nature of the reading and the exercises, some trainees simply drop out. I asked Lynn if she can tell if a volunteer is going to be any good before the investment in training.

"Not always," she said. "There have been people who seemed ideal, and they fooled me and didn't come through. And vice versa. People I wasn't sure could do it, did. In fact, there were probably more who, at first, didn't seem right, but who turned out to be great. That is because volunteers grow. They change and mature. They simply become better volunteers and better people."

And better friends.

Chapter 3

Virginia Fremont

3

VIRGINIA FREMONT

VIRGINIA FREMONT, a retired elementary schoolteacher, had lived alone most of her adult life. When her cancer progressed to the point where she knew she was dying, her younger sister, Liz, for several years a widow, moved into Virginia's little, white frame house and became her primary caregiver.

"Virginia is my inspiration," Liz said. "She's the talented one, with the education and the career."

It brought Liz great satisfaction that her sister needed her. Liz had raised six or seven children. By comparison, taking care of Virginia was almost like playing house, and she enjoyed it. She kept everything polished and shining, she fixed meals on dainty, rose-painted china, and each afternoon, she served tea.

Virginia loved the ritual of afternoon tea. Even more, she loved music. The most important thing I did for her was to go to the library for records—Chopin, Beethoven, Haydn, Rachmaninoff. I took Virginia's requests to a librarian who did everything she could to help me—so often, it seems, I discover people who want to help in every way possible.

I was needed most to run errands. I went to the pharmacy for medicine, to the food market for food, to the post office, to the library. Neither Virginia nor Liz could accept at first that they were not to pay me. When I would not accept money, they were visibly disturbed. They were very private, independent, and reserved. Accepting even the simplest things was difficult for them.

When I arrived the next time, I knew they had talked things over. When I was there, my role was to be a guest, a friend invited to tea. And tea it was—brewed freshly in a tiny, rose-painted pot and poured into those fragile little cups, biscuits from a tin, imported from England, and a tiny pot of jam. I went home hushed, almost whispering, to the amusement of my family.

"I had tea today," I said, "with two charming, cultured, lovely ladies."

One afternoon I took them a pink rose—just one—for the tea tray. For a moment Virginia's eyes glittered with tears, then we resumed our pattern of formalities and impersonal talk. I learned that day, however, that Virginia missed reading. She could not sit erect and hold a book for long, and Liz's eyes were very poor. By the next visit, I had, at the suggestion of the librarian, a recording of Robert Frost reading from his own poetry. They were delighted. The visit after that, Virginia had developed her own list of music and recorded books from those supplied by the librarian.

"Elizabeth will be able to continue with this after I am gone," she explained.

Over the next weeks, to the sounds of music and poetry, Virginia faded away. Then she died, holding Liz's hand.

Liz asked the hospice team to attend a simple memorial service she and Virginia had planned. A small group of people gathered in a little chapel of the Episcopalian church Virginia had attended before she became too ill to go out. Mostly, there was music. The minister, whom we knew as the clergyman on the team, read briefly from the Bible and offered a prayer. Then Liz reached into a florist's box lying next to her and, one at a time, took from the tissue and gave to each of us a single, white rose.

Chapter 4

Gifts

4

GIFTS

WHAT CAN A HOSPICE volunteer visiting a patient dying at home really do to help? Before I offer some of the answers that I found in my work, I want to talk about what a volunteer really cannot do—and should not try to do.

A volunteer cannot alter reality and shouldn't try. Furthermore, a volunteer cannot help at all by adding to the denial and deception that almost always surrounds terminal illness. *Terminal,* in fact, is a word people avoid, and some refuse to use it at all. That, in itself, is sometimes part of the deception.

In most people much of the time, something denies bad news. If an old and ailing relative says, "I won't be around much longer," the almost automatic response is "Nonsense!" Or worse, "You musn't talk like that!" And if the news is really bad, relatives, neighbors, even old friends simply don't find time to call or visit. It is too much of an ordeal for them, and they think they wouldn't be any good anyway. "I wouldn't know what to do." "I wouldn't know what to say."

I can listen to the words *cancer, pain, death.* And I can say them. I allow them. Sometimes my patient has been forbidden from saying them. Sometimes family members cannot talk to one another and say them. But they can talk to us, the volunteers, and we can open the door and say, "Look, your wife wants to talk to you about this. She's ready to talk about her death. Can you do this with her?"

Life-threatening cancer is very bad news. Today, fewer cancers are considered "terminal," and new hope is born every day. However, when a cancer does not respond to treatment, death is a possibility, a probability, even a certainty. When that is the case, I can go in there and make it easier, but not better. That was the big thing to learn. It is important to recognize that sometimes there is no hope even though there is life. When a person has metatases throughout his body, there is no hope—and to say there is, is fooling yourself. But to accept what is, and then to go on from there is what we do.

This is not to discredit cases of remission, even among extremely serious cases. It is to accept that among hospice cases, the really bad ones, those in the later stages of disease, remission is very rare. This is also not to be pessimistic about treatments—even cures—especially when a cancer is detected in its early stages. Truly wonderful things are happening today, and I greatly value those whose work that is. It is for me, though, to accept that the reason my patient is a hospice patient, the reason I am there at all, is that treatment is not working or has not worked in that particular case. What my patients and their families need is to become comfortable about physical care and to develop peace of mind. With them, I must face the realities of a particular life with a clear sense of mission—to help someone live the last days of his or her life to the fullest. (If a miracle is going to happen, furthermore, isn't it more likely to happen in a person who embraces life rather than in one who denies death?)

A gift of friendship helps someone live a full life. Hospice volunteers help by being friends.

- Friends accept without judgment.
- Friends recognize needs.
- Friends give time.
- Friends do what they can.

Cancer patients are found in all walks of life, all social classes, all sorts of situations. The more settings a hospice volunteer can enter, the more kinds of people she can accept, the better she can help. The gift of acceptance is rare and valuable. I think it comes from the belief that people are doing the best they know how to do to live their lives. Some are good at it, some are not so good at it, and some are just doing it differently than I would under their circumstances. As a volunteer, I need to be able to go into a home where people are doing things that I know not to do in my life. My job is not to judge; it is to see what I can do to help.

Recognizing what to do and doing it is highly personal. It depends upon the situation and the people, the chemistry of the friendship. Volunteers have different styles, strengths, and limitations; they serve in different ways. They do whatever is possible for them to do or whatever is needed—listening, sitting and talking, reading, writing, holding a hand, playing cards, watching a football game, cooking something special, washing a load of clothes, shopping for groceries, driving to the doctor's office (and keeping company for the otherwise lonely and frightening wait).

Just to be there is to help. To simply stand by can be an enormous help to a lonely patient or a member of the family who needs to get out of the house for awhile. One of my patients never even talked to me. I did absolutely nothing for her. I took something along to read, and I sat and read it—to myself. But I was helping the family to be able to go out and have a little rest from the stress of taking care of someone who is ill.

Particular experiences or education may equip volunteers to offer unique service. Della, who became involved in hospice through her Christian education experience teaching about death and dying, is particularly aware when patients are questioning their faith.

"I think all the patients at some point re-ask the question that we all ask about our faith, about God," she says. They may have asked them before, but now it's more crucial. Each life has a special and particular meaning, and a person who is dying looks over life, trying to find it."

A patient may ask, "Why do you think this has happened to me?"

Della responds, "We just don't know. This pain and suffering, this disease, is in the world, and we're part of the world, and we're not exempt from it, any of us. It isn't an easy answer. It is always easier if we can have everything mapped out to understand, but I don't think we can understand everything."

Volunteer nurses can offer professional skills: provide personal care, teach the family to perform routine care, administer medications, and answer questions troubling patients, family, and other volunteers. It is hard for me to believe that someone who works long hours in the stress-filled profession of nursing would give so freely of off-duty time. A friend, a dedicated nurse, explains why:

"It's the closeness. The fact that you can take all the time you want. You don't have to be somewhere else. No buttons popping. No buzzers buzzing. It's so nice and quiet. I can get to know a patient and really give personal care. *Personal* care."

Some patients can really use a friend to help them get something done to prepare for dying. Being able to meet certain responsibilities brings a sense of worth to a patient who could otherwise feel helpless and inadequate. Writing letters from dictation, sending out Christmas cards, organizing personal papers, paying bills—these all help a patient maintain a productive and responsible role as long as possible.

Helping to make life fuller can mean taking small gifts, especially personal ones—homemade cookies, homegrown flowers, homemade chicken soup, tomatoes from a home garden. Helping someone to live fully may also mean accepting small gifts—a cutting from a houseplant, a division of a perennial, a favorite family recipe.

I send valentines, Easter cards, friendship cards, birthday cards—mail is important and holidays are important. I gave one poor soul the only Christmas gifts she got on her last Christmas, a poinsettia and a soft flannel nightgown. One patient asked me to help her give what she knew was going to be her last birthday party. I put eighty candles on her cake and burned myself lighting them. She loved it.

Good volunteers—volunteers who do the most

good—are simply good friends, willing to help without intruding and ready to respond to simple, human needs. Even sort of peculiar ones ....

One of the best things I ever did for a patient was to stand by her cats. First, I do not like cats. And hers were spoiled rotten. But she positively adored them, and her greatest fear was that something awful would happen to them. I found out, not surprisingly, that no one wanted two old, spoiled cats, who could not (of course!) be separated. Just in time, I found a veterinarian and saint who lived on a farm, who gave his word that he would take them. When she died—and believe me, those cats knew it—I had to catch them, and .... Well, I did it. It was what she wanted.

Sometimes the patient needs very little, while someone else in the family is in desperate need of a caring friend.

Fred, only 45, had become comatose before I started—that was early in June. I could do nothing for him. At the end of May his teenage son had been killed in a car accident after a drinking party. The 12-year sister blamed their parents for her brother's death. And, she deeply resented my being there. While I understood her reactions to be normal, there was nothing I could do for her, she so completely closed me out. I could offer support, however, for her mother Nancy. Nancy would be waiting when I came. She would fall into my arms and ask me to sit with her on the porch. She would talk and talk and talk—for the whole three hours I was there. Most of all, she needed me to listen.

Nancy really needed to unload. People she thought were friends shied away because too many "bad things" had happened to that family. Working two part-time jobs besides, she had almost no time or opportunity for talk. No one shared with her the heavy pain of her son's death, the burden of her husband's illness, and the dread of more to come.

"Oh, God!" she said. "I have not even been allowed to grieve for that boy."

To be there when the words are ready to come, shyly, in a whisper, or surging like flood waters, or rambling on and on, to be there to listen is the greatest gift of all. To listen, openly, without judgment, without advice, without interruption, without finishing sentences—to hear.

An anonymous poem we were given during our training left a lasting impression on me. It began like this:

"When I ask you to listen to me and you start giving me advice, you have not done what I asked.

When I ask you to listen to me and you begin to tell me why I shouldn't feel that way, you are trampling on my feelings.

When I ask you to listen to me and you feel you

have to do something to solve my problems, you have failed me ...

Listening allows one who needs to talk to stay in control, intact, and whole—to do what needs to be done to work things out:

"And I can do for myself. I'm not helpless. Maybe discouraged and faltering, but not helpless.

When you do something for me that I can and need to do for myself, you contribute to my fear and inadequacy ...

So please listen and just hear me."

People who are dying also need someone to listen because listening affirms their lives. Listening allows them to make gifts to us of their thoughts, feelings, and experiences. Out of these we form our memories, our memories shape our lives, and we share our memories when they promise to be of value. Life, in that way, goes on.

Chapter 5

Emma Gruber

5

EMMA GRUBER

EMMA GRUBER was a big, broad, heavy-boned woman, full of salt and vinegar, invincible, somehow, even as she was dying. She wanted to die in her own home, and she really liked the hospice way. To qualify, however, Emma needed a primary caregiver—someone who would be in her home as a key contact person for the program. Capable as ever at solving the problems of everyday living, she placed an ad, conducted interviews, and hired a housekeeper.

From the start, Emma and I liked one another. I loved her spunk and spirit, and I know I just lit up when I went there. Visiting Emma made my day, maybe because we were sort of on the same wave length. We were real friends in no time. And our friendship became a family-like relationship. My husband visited Emma—the only time he ever met with a patient—and he liked her instantly.

Emma's disease progressed, yet she met each challenge as it came. Chemotherapy, she believed, was making her unnecessarily sick. So she called her doctor.

"Let's face it," she said, "I'm dying and nothing is going to change that. So I have decided to discontinue my treatments."

She had a young doctor who was fond of her and who admired her. He evidently protested because next she said, "It's all right. You've done a wonderful job. Now don't feel responsible, because it's my decision. It's my body."

That apparently took care of it. Then, she turned to me and said, "It is so hard on a doctor to lose a patient. They are trained to save lives, you know. They work so hard to keep you alive. I hope he doesn't feel he's failed."

One morning, when the housekeeper Blanche was in the laundry out of earshot, Emma got out of bed and broke her leg. She felt it and heard it break—her pain must have been excrutiating. Clear-headed and clever, she dialed Operator on her bedside phone.

"I'm having trouble with my phone. I'm going to hang up, and I want you to dial me back." And she gave her number.

When the phone rang and Blanche heard the operator's strange message, she knew it was Emma who was trying to call her.

Although Emma fully accepted the fact that she was dying, when she returned from the hospital in a wheelchair, she said to me with the deepest sadness, "I don't think I'm ever going to walk again. Sally, do you realize what that means—never to walk again!"

We became still closer in our relationship—seldom is a patient-volunteer relationship so intense. We were like mother and daughter sometimes, like sisters other times, always friends. Seldom, too, does a case extend for so long a period. Nine months. While that may seem a short time to develop a deep bond, it is a great deal of time when none of it is wasted.

Emma really opened up and let me in. I don't believe she had ever before allowed herself the luxury of talking all she wanted to. She told me all about her life, her mistakes, her disappointments, and her triumphs. She *used* me in the best possible way, accepting with open arms everything I had to give. I felt myself grow stronger as she became weaker. She gave me rich memories, deep and lasting images of a noble spirit, bigger than life.

When she died, she died in my arms. I did not take another case for a month.

Chapter 6

Rewards

6

REWARDS

WHILE IT IS TRUE that volunteers are not paid, in money, that is, they receive as much as they give. There are various and complex needs that hospice volunteer work gratifies. The rewards, although not guaranteed, are nevertheless great. They are things like self-esteem, fulfillment, personal growth, insight, even enlightenment.

I am a realist, and hard-nosed. I know I do this work to get something out of it. And, I'm not ashamed to say so. I began to feel rewarded even before I worked with patients. The training was good for me. The woman who conducted our training, Lynn Abram, is one of the more outstanding people who ever touched my life. She is bright, sensitive, kind, gentle, just about everything that a person should be. She gave us an intense, ten-day training that was one of the best things that I have ever done.

I would come home every night and say, "I'm not sure I can ever help someone to die, but the training that I am getting is making me a better person. It is making me more sensitive to people's needs, not only to those of dying people."

Some of my own most important needs are fulfilled in this work. I need to comfort. I need to be needed. More than that, I need to be needed for what I, in particular, can give. I want to be invited in through doors held open by those who need help. And I like to be invited all the way in.

The design and operation of a program is important to consider when talking about rewards. In any volunteer situation, it is possible to be exploited and mistreated. Even though there is no paycheck, there *are* working conditions, coworkers, supervisors, and policies. Volunteer work is, after all, work. It matters how things are done and how people behave toward one another.

It is personally rewarding to be respected by the professional people involved in the hospice program. I work among the finest nurses, doctors, and clergy as a valued team member. When we discuss a case at a team meeting and my insight about something is recognized, for example, I feel I have contributed what I, and no one else, can. Our hospice places a high value on its volunteers. Lay volunteers and clergy are valued by everybody, including the paid skilled workers. That was clear from the start.

I remember well the training session that began, "This program depends upon a full set of mutually satisfactory relationships."

Since everyone knows the volunteers are important, we have the support we need to perform well. Although not professionals, volunteers are trained for the job and develop their skills through experience. We are not "amateurs," except in the sense that we must not accept money for our work. And, we gain "professional" satisfaction in using our skills and being valued for our work.

Rewarding friendships form among people who work together and come to respect one another's work. These friendships are very often highly successful, rich and lasting, because of the commonality of both experience and values. I have made close friends through this work. That's not surprising when you consider the kind of experiences we have shared.

One experience really stands out. Two of us volunteers were sent to the same house at the same time to babysit. We had been briefed, of course, so we knew there were several children there. The home was rather off the beaten path in a rural area, so it was nice to have company. Pat, who was my partner, is a nurse. That made sense because one of the children was a serious diabetic who would need an insulin shot. Still, two volunteers at once?

Once we were there, babies and children seemed to be everywhere. And, right in the middle of it all, an old woman lay dying of cancer.

Martha, the woman who held all this together, and alone, usually, was running almost a hospice orphanage of her own. She made room for any child who needed a place to be, and the old woman as well. The dining room table was outfitted as a changing table, for instance, with fresh, folded laundry piled neatly down one side. The old woman's medicines were lined up high on a book shelf near her bed, out of reach of little fingers, next to an alarm clock. A time chart was taped to the wall.

The babies were beautifully cared for and very happy, but they were also very active! It took the two of us running constantly to keep some kind of order. By the end of the afternoon we were friends. We still are.

There is a distinction between giving one's time and giving one's self, and the rewards vary accordingly. Doing work, simply because it must be done, can be satisfying and worthwhile. The time itself is certainly a gift, and a costly one these days. On the other hand, being recognized as someone special—someone particularly sensitive, for example, or trustworthy—is a different thing. It is not selfless, it is full of self, and that makes a difference in its quality. For me, and probably for most of us, volunteer work can be disappointingly unrewarding when that quality is lacking. That happens sometimes. It is sometimes hard to remember that the patient's needs are more important than one's own. Learning that can be a hard lesson.

The least satisfying experience I have had was with a man I'll call Francis. He wouldn't let me do my thing. Through Francis' door flowed what seemed an endless stream of people from his church and men from a lodge he belonged to. They came carrying food of all kinds and filling the refrigerator to brimming. They sent so many flowers the house looked as though he had already died. In a way, these people were the return on Francis' investment: he had spent almost all his spare time in good works.

Francis let me give him his medicine, he let me make his lunch, he let me make up a chart of who came or called and when, and he let me address his thank-you cards. He let me, that is, if I thought to ask. He asked me only for the most superficial things in the most formal voice.

"Lower the shade a little, if you please. That's perfect. You're a big help."

Anyone could have done those things. I could have been anyone. I was not useful to him as myself. I was an appliance. He did not need *me,* and he would not let me show him that I could give him more.

With Francis I didn't get that feeling that I had helped to make it easier for him. I feel, instead, an emptiness about him. He didn't really give me, didn't give hospice, a chance. He didn't level with us. In the end, he took his physical complaints to his personal physician, for instance, not to his hospice team. Francis' doctor had no choice but to send him to the hospital, into surgery, and prescribe drugs that eased his pain by making him comatose. And, his dying dragged on. Eventually he died alone in the hospital.

We could have made it better for Francis if only he had let us. I know that. But I also know that I must not, in fact, I cannot, force caring and comfort on one who doesn't want it. It is still hard for me to keep in mind the lesson this man had to teach me. As my patient, Francis was absolutely within his rights to do things his way. He had the right to be impersonal towards me. He also had the right to reject hospice. He is the one who counted.

One dear old gentleman, Paul, once a heavy smoker, was debilitated by inoperable lung cancer. He suffered almost as much from his regrets. He had left home very young, ignoring his parents' repeated attempts to bring him back, he married and had a son, and the marriage ended in divorce. He lost touch with both families, his mother and father, his wife and son. His parents died suddenly in a car crash. He had never written to his son.

The poor man couldn't rest. He wanted to get all this off his chest, and he knew it was safe to tell me. He had never told any of this to his wife (his second wife for about thirty years), a lovely woman who thought he was wonderful.

There was something in him that really touched me. I saw a man who had tried, had failed, and had finally got it together. I admired him for that, I told him. And I admired him for the concern, and love, he felt for his parents and his son, even though he had been unable to express it or act on it in any way. I know I helped by just listening and, in a way, forgiving him. I know it had something to do with my being the mother of two sons. I felt needed for the same kind of skill at listening, without judgment, to someone using me to work things out.

He was very, very weak. I took a chance and urged him to write a letter to his son, and then I helped him to write it, and I mailed it for him. After he did that, he told his wife everything. She was wonderful.

"All these years, I knew there was something," she told me. "Poor man. What an awful burden."

He died soon afterward. Really peacefully, I think. Sometime later, his wife called me to say she had heard from the son. He really appreciated his father's letter, and he was sorry he hadn't written in time. (That's ironic, isn't it?) I feel good about that case. I know I made a difference. I was a real friend to that whole family.

To be needed. To make a difference. These are the

rewards. Occasionally, even rarely, can a volunteer make so much difference. Most often, it is little contributions that continue to reinforce a feeling of value. What comes back seems so much greater than what is given.

What I get is a lot of appreciation. I get a lot more back than I give. And I really give mothering, mothering complete with chicken soup. I make good chicken soup—with a pinch of dill in it. For every cup of chicken soup I take with me, I come home with a gallon. One dear lady, for instance, died a few months after I started visiting her. For her ninetieth birthday I baked a little chocolate cake and took her an African violet, and her brother and I sang "Happy Birthday" for her.

"Thank you for my birthday party," she said. "You know this is my last one. You have made it a very special one." Just before she died, she said, "Thank you for being here with me. You made me not afraid to die."

Her last meal on earth was my chicken soup.

Chapter 7

Arthur Wilcox

7

ARTHUR WILCOX

HAD ARTHUR WILCOX been my first case, I wonder if I would have gone on volunteering. This case was not typical, but to leave it out would make my account unrealistic. When people ask me how I do it, I think of Arthur Wilcox.

"Sometimes I don't."

Arthur was a poor soul dying in a dirty and dispirited house. There was nothing I could do to change that. I tried. We all tried, but nothing would give. When I look back I realize that it was not my fault or the fault of the hospice team; it was not the failure of the hospice concept. It was a tough case, that's all.

Arthur just sat, and stared off or at the television set, and whimpered about one thing or another, and I just sat with him so his daughter Gwen could go out for awhile. Arthur was fully conscious, alert, able to get about a little on his own, but he was totally placid. There was nothing he wanted to do, or try, or hear about, or talk about. He just sat, a lump in a bed. I ran very quickly out of suggestions.

Gwen, Arthur's daughter, considered her father nothing but a weight dumped onto her life by her mother who had suddenly died of a heart attack—and for that she would never forgive her. She deliberately forgot her. And Robert, Gwen's husband, just completely forgot his father-in-law.

"Who? Oh, that. Just keep me out of that." With his hand he swatted at the thought of him, as if at a gnat, and walked away from all of it.

Sunlight turned murky as it passed through stiff curtains smelling of rust and stale cigarettes. The humid air that oppressive summer coated everything inside with stickiness. The atmosphere was thick with heat and unhappiness. Gwen's two skinny little boys hung around whining and bickering until sent out "to play," something they could not do without making their dog wail.

I sat with Arthur several times while Gwen went out "for food." The house needed food. The refrigerator held only beer and cheap pop, and the kitchen shelves, almost nothing. Gwen brought back fried chicken or pizza. The only other "fresh" food I saw was open boxes of donuts. I took Arthur soup and fruit—none of which he even wanted to try. The most I ever saw him eat was half an egg. He was literally wasting away.

To make things worse Gwen and Arthur had never liked one another. Arthur's dying only made it worse.

Gwen had married young, and not very well, "just to get away from home." Gwen did not want her father in her home either, and she showed it by neglecting him terribly. She never heard him call, she never thought about opening his window or turning on his fan. But she did hear her father's television set when her own wasn't on.

And then she shrieked, "Turn that damn thing down!"

We held a team conference every week. On this case we had two nurses, a social worker, and an attending physician. Everyone was frustrated, and I thought, too patient. Arthur wasn't kept clean, he didn't get his medications unless one of us visited at the right time, and he was starving.

"That woman should be reported to the Board of Health!" I remember saying.

Then I began to develop what I thought was a nervous reaction to that household, a terrible prickling sensation, first around my ankles, then all over my legs. My case of "nerves" turned out to be flea bites, and I asked to be taken off the case.

Arthur went to a nursing home.

Chapter 8

Perspectives

8

PERSPECTIVES

"HOW DO YOU DO IT!" friends and family say.

"I just do it."

I don't just do it. That's not a serious answer. It wasn't a serious question, either. The real question is, how does a volunteer, an ordinary everyday person, face willingly and repeatedly what society perceives to be a morbid danger? Terminal cancer is one of the terrors of our times.

First of all, I know I cannot die from contact with either cancer or death—I can't "catch" it. A surprising number of people think one can, at least at some superstitious, what-you-know-can-hurt-you level. (It is realistic, on the other hand, to say I can die from smoke and flames if I volunteer to fight fires.) Being realistic about the danger is important.

I do have to cope with the stress of being around pain and suffering. I do have to cope with the strain of everybody's feelings, the raw nerves, the sadness, the grief, the fear, the anger, the resentment. And the way I look at it is to remember that what works for the living works for the dying. I do it the same way I do everything else:

I can learn what I can, I get support if I can, then I trust what I know about living.

A good hospice program provides a structure of knowledge and support so a volunteer doesn't get swallowed up in the work. A good program carefully selects volunteer trainees, as I've said before, and training further selects as well as prepares them. Not everyone stays on, remember. Although training varies from program to program, a good program can be expected to provide certain things.

- It will focus on the hospice concept and the local interpretation of that concept. While hospice provides comfort and care when nothing more medically can be done to change the course of the disease, it takes a variety of forms in a variety of settings.
- It will provide a highly personal orientation to services and personnel—providing speakers, for instance, from its own professional staff as well as its veteran volunteers.
- It will teach a great deal about cancer—its kinds, symptoms, stages.
- It will teach about death—its stages, its processes, its signs.
- It will teach even more about the terminal cancer

patient's emotional reaction to the disease—to changes in body functioning, to sexuality, to sensuality.

• And, it will teach a volunteer how to help, how to manage stress, grief and loss. How to manage physical and emotional pain. How to relieve pain, sometimes.

My training was excellent, as I've said several places. I learned lessons about myself and others that will serve me my whole life. I got my best training at home, though. My mother showed me how to care. I remember when my father was dying, and he had become a thin, frail shell, so fragile, so still. We didn't know if he could see us or hear us, or even know if we were there. My mother lay down softly alongside him and took him in her arms. She just held him close for a long, long time. He was her man. She loved him.

Experience continues the teaching process. A good program will attempt to shape the experience of volunteers in order to provide opportunities for greater skill and personal growth.

• **First, a good program will carefully match a volunteer to a case.**

"You have to know what your volunteers like to do and don't like to do," Lynn Abram explains. "You get to know who can go where, who can stand smells, who needs a clean house, who needs a talker...." Some volunteers are comfortable and effective in almost any setting. However, she adds, "Depressing, distressing, difficult hospice cases or settings require especially careful selection of volunteers."

She had a real knack for knowing who to send where. She knew who could handle what stress or moral issues, for instance. Everybody is faint-hearted or weak-kneed about something. Some people could not be given a home where there had been a suicide. Someone who will "stick up her nose" cannot go to a home where there is an illegitimate child.

When I began, I knew right away that I could not work with children. (Lynn asked all of us whether there were some kind of patient that we didn't think we could handle.) While I knew some people would be great with kids, I said, "I just don't think I could do that."

I must add a postscript to this now and to what I said about growing as a volunteer. Today, I work at Pittsburgh's wonderful Children's Hospital with children who have cancer. Yes, it is very, very sad, sometimes. And, yes, I love what I am doing there.

- **Then, after a careful assignment is made, a good hospice program will prepare a volunteer for the specific case.**

I am given every inch of available information. I am told the name of the patient, the age of the patient, the diagnosis, the duration of the illness, any complications, the doctor, the medication, the side effects (for instance, loss of hair with chemotherapy). I am told the name of the primary caregiver (the key contact person at home), the relationship of the caregiver, the amount and kind of stress in the family, the reaction and attitude of the other family members. (It often happens, for instance, that young children are resentful of illnesses in their home.) And, I am given the names and functions of the other members of the team. I always make it a point to call the registered nurse assigned to the case because she is usually very tuned in.

- **Finally, a good program will provide support to see a volunteer through a case.**

In my situation there are team conferences every other week, more, if needed (remember Arthur?). They include the hospice nurse (a registered nurse professional), the medical director, the volunteer or volunteers, the social worker, and the clergy person, if there is one. We all give our input. We give one another suggestions. We share the stress. We help one another become more effective.

I once had a patient in terrible, intractable pain. Although her pain was beyond what we could manage at home, she did not want to go to a hospital and be drugged. She was more afraid of unconsciousness than of pain, I guess. I couldn't stand how much she was hurting. And she wasn't dying! At the team conference I asked our medical director to tell me, please, when she would die. That question is downright unethical. So is an answer.

Carefully, gently, the doctor replied, "Sally, most patients who are in the situation this patient is in don't last very long."

That was so reassuring to me. That helped me keep going where I was needed.

Occasionally a situation can become very tough for anyone to handle. In those cases, team conferences can save the case. Lynn explains:

"In a really difficult situation, where difficult family members divide the team up, setting one hospice person against another, for instance, or where very manipulative patients tell the volunteer one thing, the nurse another, that sort of thing, we hold additional conferences, so that the team will be cohesive towards that family. This doesn't happen often. Nice families are the rule."

Once in a while, though, something has to give ....

I was in a home, once, where I just, well, here's what happened. This sweet man lay dying of colon cancer. His wife was recovering from very minor surgery. He liked talking to me. Meanwhile, his wife kept interrupting with horrible stories about him. She was a real shrew.

She turned on him, "Look at him! He's disgusting.

He really picked a great time to die!" Then she turned on me. She accused me of trying to steal him away from her—and she really meant it.

There are a lot of complicated reasons for behavior like that. It was in a team conference, trying to unscramble the thing, that we decided a male volunteer would work out better, and we took me off the case.

A good program, then, gets a volunteer off to a good start. Once you have that, asking "How do you do it?" is asking what personal resources a volunteer draws upon to do this work from day to day. To do this work, or any work, here's what I think you need:

- **You have to know yourself.**

You have to know who you are. If you are a mother, you mother. If you are a nurse, you provide nursing care. Down deep, you know your style. You know when you are being yourself. And don't try to be what you are not.

Most of us, I think, are good at being good friends. From friendly neighbors to close friends of the family. Good friends know how to work on a friendship. We do the things for hospice patients that we do for other people. We think about them, think about what will make a visit good for them. Then we take along a story to tell, a pack of cards, snapshots, a suggestion, a jar of jam, some flowers, a poem. Mostly, I take with me a sense of their need. I stay open to what has to be done. And, I do it. I've learned this about my life: somehow, what I need to do, I do.

- **You have to take care of yourself.**

You have to be good to yourself, first. You have to look after your needs. Only then is there enough left over to give away. I reward myself. I treat myself. I am very, very good to me. I never feel selfish, and if I am selfish, that's fine. Hospice is part of this. Hospice is good for me.

Della sees it a little bit differently, "One thing I've learned is that it is very necessary for me to take some time just for myself. I swim three times a week. And I pull apart—I like to be by myself—and read. There was a point where I felt that was a selfish thing, but I recognize that I can only give, even to my family, if I take time to be by myself and to take *in* to myself."

- **You have to have realistic expectations.**

Like knowing you cannot make it better—you cannot make cancer go away. What you can do is offer comfort and friendship to patient and family. Like realizing that if a family is a mess, someone's cancer will only make it more so—and it's not your fault. You can, though, relieve some of the stress on a family. Like accepting that people don't always choose what's good for them. They are doing the best they can. You can only keep offering the best you have.

- **You have to know how to shift gears.**

Life is full of sadness and humor, time to work, time to unwind. Hospice work means putting some things behind while you do other things—like forgetting for awhile that you are having twenty-eight people to Thanksgiving dinner. If you allow yourself to get rattled about that, you can't, for instance, feed a patient slowly, calmly, one of a few tiny meals that give him a little pleasure.

You have to know how to "make" time, to juggle the pursuits and demands of family, self and others—and make it all work.

- **You have to know your limitations.**

I cannot do this work continuously. Some people can. I take breaks, especially if I have become very involved, as I did after Emma Gruber died, when I took a month off. I also won't take more than one patient at a time. Some people do. I know a man who has four cases right now. That would not be good for me.

- **You have to know how to let go.**

After a patient dies, I follow up with cards and phone calls, a common practice among volunteers. The connection fades, gradually, usually, until we finally lose contact. At some point people seem just not to need the connection anymore. I may get the feeling that they have had all they want of me, that I am just a painful reminder, so I accept that and just let go.

Occasionally there are longer ties. There are hospice volunteers, I'm sure, who have literally become members of a patient's family. But I have to be able to separate myself and get on with my life. I'm not sure that everyone feels that way, but I do, and I feel strongly about it. I have to get on with the next thing.

I may even have to let go of this work, to move on to something else. I do things in cycles. If, or when, it is time to change, to grow another way, I feel it and go on. I knew when it was time to do hospice work, I knew when it was time to work with children with cancer, and I may move on to something else. It is 0.K. to be finished with something. Perhaps to come back. Perhaps not.

- **You have to love life.**

I almost neglected to add this until a friend pointed out what I guess I take for granted. If you love life, thoroughly, you want to know all about it. So you follow it to its end. Most of all, you have to be sure that anyone who is coming to the end of it, if you have a thing to say or do about it, is living every last moment to its fullest.

She's right. And I intend to live every last moment of my own life to its fullest.

Chapter 9

Mr. Miller

9

MR. MILLER

IMAGINE a sprawling ranch house with huge sparkling windows through which, in any room, you see trees and flowers, children and dogs. Imagine the dining room, with fireplace, a view of the patio—and in the middle, surrounded by three adorable little boys, an old, white-haired man dying of cancer. That's the way Mr. Miller thought it was supposed to be. For him, it was.

Mr. Miller, as his daughter-in-law Sarah addressed him (and so, of course, did I), was a widower who lived by himself until his cancer presented a choice, not whether to accept nursing care, but what kind. He was weakening; he needed a wheelchair to get around and help to climb into it. In his case, chemotherapy didn't seem to do anything but make him sick and take more and more of his hair.

Once it was clear that his father was probably dying of cancer, Richard Miller thought the only choice was a nursing home or a hospital. He thought it would be "better for everyone" if his father were hospitalized. Mr. Miller did not want either—he was adamant. And Sarah wouldn't hear of it.

When Sarah suggested that her father-in-law move in, Richard said, "I can't ask you to do that."

"I'm asking you to please let me," Sarah said.

So Mr. Miller moved into the dining room.

Family life did not stop or even slow down. During the day the phone rang constantly, people visited, the radio played while Sarah took care of the house, and she and Mr. Miller had lunch and a talk. After school, the boys headed for the bed in the dining room, to tell what happened, to show papers, and to chase their puppy from the bed and around the circle from dining room, to kitchen, to family room, to living room, and back to dining room. In the evening, father and son talked.

I was there twice, the first time to stay with the boys while Sarah took Mr. Miller for chemotherapy. When I got there, a plumber was in the kitchen, the phone was ringing, and the boys, like baby bears, were rolling around the floor. Sarah, cool and capable, was checking over a list of notes she had for me, so I would "feel comfortable." Mr. Miller was neatly dressed and ready to go. He explained to me in detail how Sarah had designed and constructed "all by herself," a clever little ramp that helped her get the wheelchair from the porch to the walk and from the walk to the driveway.

"It is a pleasure to have such a wonderful daughter-in-law," he said.

"Sally, he is a very special man," Sarah said.

The second time I was there, to babysit while Sarah went out, I saw a marked difference in Mr. Miller. He was fading. His skin was as white as his hair had been. Most of his hair was gone. He was as delicate as porcelain with fine blue lines and shadows. He smiled slowly and reached his hand no more than an inch above the bed, but I knew it was a salute to my being there. Even the bears and the puppy seemed to feel his fragility. They were almost subdued.

The next week, the evening before I was to make my third visit, Sarah called.

"Sally, we all want to be alone tomorrow," she said. "I know you will understand. Mr. Miller is very, very close. And we want to say good-bye, by being there as a family."

I almost asked her to say good-bye for me too, but I thought better of it and simply said, "I do understand."

Mr. Miller died quietly, early in the afternoon.

Chapter 10

Choices

10

CHOICES

I HAVE TRIED to reach a number of people with this book: potential hospice volunteers and potential hospice families, in particular. I have tried to give a sense of having been there through my experience. It is *experience* I have tried to provide, more than the usual *information* available through hospitals and libraries.

I have only touched upon certain issues that by now are likely to concern anyone who has read this far. I have focused upon the details of relationship and interaction among people, not upon symptoms, techniques, arrangements, routines. Neither have I provided specific details about care; I have instead shown that because hospice is a team effort, there are hands, and shoulders, and hearts enough to give care—specialized nursing care as well as tender human care.

Before I close, however, there is a piece of the picture I want to highlight—the matter of *choice.*

To make a choice, one must have, recognize, and exercise options. For the dying person, there is the choice of hospice or hospital, a choice that is not always clear. Too often a family sees one of its members as under sentence of death and the future as without alternatives. Those of us who don't simply die suddenly without warning may get sent to the hospital to die—that is all too commom practice. It may seem more efficient and more manageable, even though the family has to make trips to the hospital and sit on uncomfortable chairs, sometimes interminably. Close family members will feel guilty when they cannot be there, even as they carry on the necessary routines of their lives, knowing the dying person is left alone.

Although the hospice movement is growing, people eligible for hospice die lonely or drugged deaths in hospitals. Tragically, the emphasis is placed upon their dying, not upon their living their last days as fully as possible.

People who have heard of hospice may dismiss it without serious consideration, as something out of the question. Or something only other people do. Perhaps the patient thinks, "I couldn't ask my family to let me die at home. I don't want to be a burden." Or the person who would be responsible for providing most of the care thinks, "I am not up to that. I just don't have the strength, I don't have the patience, I'm not the type." Or the adult child of a dying parent sees hospice as a burden falling on a partner and the experience as bad for children,

"I can't ask my wife to take care of my father ...."

It is not unusual for families, as well as patients, to deny illness and the possibility of death. It is true today that many cancers are not terminal if they are caught and treated early. When there is little or no reason to hope for a reprieve, however, a family's refusal to accept death as a possibility may also mean a family's refusal to accept it—and the benefits of a hospice program.

Denial can run the gamut from blaming the patient for somehow making up a phony disease to believing recovery is just outside the door waiting to come in. Some families will say a patient isn't dying, when the patient *is* dying. They will say he's getting better, when he *is not* getting better. They will say he seems better, he looks better, it is just a matter of time before he will be much better .... So they never consider what hospice could do.

Life is by definition terminal. The trick is living it—all of it. Denial is a curse when it means we ignore an illness, as if ignoring it will send it away. Instead, we need to pay very close attention *to the patient* and do the things that matter—while there is time. It is true that denial can bring strength to those patients who use it to fight illness. Some win. They draw from denial the energy to get the most out of opportunities for living, which, in their case include treatments. Those who are beyond the reach of treatment draw from their *acceptance of death* a similar energy to take full advantage of their own opportunities for living.

Occasionally the family pressures the doctor to provide treatment, and more treatment, when treatment isn't working. Doctors aim to heal, and failing that, to do no harm. When healing does not happen, the doctor may be pressured to "do something" and so do something harmful. Continuous chemotherapy or radiation, and surgery—performing surgery to set a bone, for example, in a body that will never heal—can sometimes make a dying patient sicker and weaker needlessly.

A doctor may recommend hospice care, and many do. A doctor may also have no choice but to hospitalize a patient when the patient and family cannot choose among alternatives. A doctor cannot spend hours counseling a family thrown into confusion by a diagnosis of terminal cancer. Leaving too much "up to the doctor," too, will probably mean hospitalization. How else can a doctor manage to see that care is provided? A doctor's role is not to minister to the dying, although some do. It may be more convenient for the doctor to hospitalize a patient because the doctor is not trained, comfortable, or equipped to deal with terminal care.

Early in my experience with hospice, I learned that however "efficient," hospitalization can be devastating for patient and family. I visited a woman, Betty, only twice. The second time, one week after my first visit, I was shocked at the difference in her. She was despondent and depressed, her eyes were dull, her smile was gone, her skin was floury. Her medicine, I thought, is draining her. The next day Betty's daughter called and told me that the doctor wanted to adjust her medicine in the hospital where he could watch her.

"My mother became hysterical," she told me. "I'll never forget the way she said, 'I do not want to go in the hospital. I know I'm going to die. I do not want to die there.' "

Later that day, I got a phone call. "She died, Sally," Betty's daughter said. "She didn't want to die in the hospital. And, I never got to say goodbye." Her heart was broken.

Families may reject the hospice alternative out of fear of death. Families who choose hospice, however, also wrestle with fear of death. The difference is that hospice prepares a family for death as no traditional hospital service can hope to.

If a family fears the approach of death and is caught in a dreadful anticipation of loss, hospice can relieve some of the tension and anxiety with constructive work. As patients grow weaker and weaker, as time goes on, a family can begin its process of grief. Death is not the shock that it is otherwise. Helen, after her father had died years before in a nursing home, took care of her mother at home.

"I knew all the time my mother was dying that I was doing what I could. I was there. I knew I had chosen not to send her away. And, afterwards, there was much less upset, less guilt."

If a family fears the actual moment of death, hospice can counteract that fear with a plan for coping. It seems that the actual death could be a problem, but it is not. From training and experience, I know most of the time patients drift away in their sleep. Regardless, the nurse assigned to the case or the volunteer tells the family what to expect—and on a patient-by-patient basis, what to expect is not too hard to predict. Because everyone is so well prepared, the moment of death is not a hysterical moment for the family. And following death, there's a system of steps to put into operation. The first is to call the hospice office, a 24-hour number which is right at hand.

Fears about death, like most fears, are forms of the greatest fears of all, fear of the unknown. They can be relieved by knowledge. There are more. Recognizing these fears may help a patient or a family to make, rather than avoid making, a choice.

• Fear of pain. Fear of suffering or watching while someone suffers.

It is a common misconception that pain is more manageable in a hospital, or too serious to deal with at home, or too hard for a family to take.

There is less pain than most people realize. Some patients, it is true, suffer intractable pain. Some have no pain. What pain there is, is usually manageable with special techniques, such as deep-breathing exercises and medications that quiet pain while the patient stays alert and his mind stays sharp. Busy hospitals may be unable to work closely with a patient in gaining control over his pain; they may have no choice but to drug him into virtual unconsciousness.

• Fear of upheaval.

Stress, tension, sadness—these things are expected and are made easier with the kind of support system hospice offers.

A man fighting bone cancer has agreed to move from his two-bedroom, two-story home to a one-floor, two-bedroom apartment in the same neighborhood. By not separating himself off by steps, he will be able to stay part of everyday life much better, and his wife will have an easier time providing care at home.

Perhaps a patient has to move in from somewhere else, how does the average family find or make the room?

We don't all have spare bedrooms, to be sure, but bedrooms are not the only places in which to die. In the case of Mr. Miller, a young woman turned the dining room into a wonderful room for her father-in-law. He liked being right in the middle of the family, right near the kitchen. It is not unusual to do things this way.

- Fear of weakness. Fear of being unable to cope. Fear of being unable to manage, not knowing how to meet the needs of a dying patient.

It is important to remember that coping is learned, that hospice exists to provide the learning and support needed to manage. (Not being there may be harder to handle.) I wasn't sure I could do hospice work when I started. I don't expect a family to feel competent at first at providing care. That's why the hospice team is there. And the team is made up of people who can help a particular family. One family may need more than one volunteer, one a psychiatric social worker, one close involvement with a clergy person. One dear lady who had lost a great amount of weight, was very embarrassed that her dentures no longer fit, so we found her a dentist who made house calls. We all work together to make it possible to manage—to make it go much, much better than otherwise.

Tragically, out of ignorance, denial, fear, pride, or a combination of those, some families never learn the difference hospice could make, and it could make all the difference in the world.

It is important to make the choice as soon as there is reason to believe a cancer could be terminal and death inevitable. Hospice care can and often should begin before a patient is bedridden. Patients who have small or busy families, for instance, may need tangible things like transportation to and from a doctor. Over time, and as the disease progresses, a relationship between the patient and a volunteer has a chance to develop and then deepen. Like friends, they can enjoy lunch out, a movie, a concert, and some long talks, perhaps. As death draws closer and the emotional as well as the tangible needs increase, a strong system has been created to meet them.

Unfortunately, sometimes a family chooses hospice so late that so little support is possible. It is far better to make contact early. It is so sad when we get a patient who has only a week or so of life left. One visit is hardly enough to make a difference. The family is hit much harder, too, with regrets and guilt.

EPILOGUE

TO THOSE FACING A CHOICE—whether to serve as a volunteer or to choose hospice as a way of life when dying is certain—I pass along these words from an address by an oncologist to a group of volunteers in training.

The speaker is Robert Hilberg, a doctor who knows the difference hospice can make.

I continue to be tremendously impressed, even amazed, at what in a relatively short time hospice can do for patients who are trying to live while they die.

I see a sequence that seems to happen—if there is enough time.

First, there is a period of settling in, during which all concerned learn comfort about giving and reach a peace of mind about the physical aspects of care.

When the patient and the patient's family achieve peace of mind, when they settle in, when they become more comfortable with the fact that they can in a very competent fashion with your help deliver physical care, this will allow the luxury of deeper questions.

Then is a time of asking "What are you thinking?" "Are you afraid?" "What are you feeling?" "What kind of hope do you have?" "What kind of hope is left?" "Have you lost it?" "What's good, what's bad, about the past, about now?" "Are there things that need to be said that you'd like to say?"

I'll listen.

I'll hear.

I'll watch.

I'll see.

When that comfortable time comes and when you can share in reflections, don't forget the children. The children can never be too young, and never too old, to share in the care, to share in the feelings. They can provide something they will later remember and cherish—an ability to comfort a person they love.

Don't let the children spend the rest of their lives wishing they could have said, "I know you, Mother. I love you."

If you have done these things, then the time to go away will be sad. That time will be painful. If you have been good, the leaving will be hard. You need to remember what was built and to take joy in what was given. That person will live in your thoughts and your reflections with the family.

A special thing happened.

You built a leaving, a going away that was full and meaningful, not empty. You gave the finest thing at the hardest time of life.

So cry.

But then smile.

And then laugh.

RESOURCES

Information about local hospice programs is available from hospitals—just by calling and asking for the hospice office. Usually hospice care must be requested by physicians; however, *referrals can be initiated by patients, family members, clergy, even friends.* Hospice home care is ordinarily less expensive than traditional hospital care; furthermore, medical insurance covers most hospice programs.

Information concerning hospice care and volunteerism is also available at local university medical libraries and national organization home offices.

General Information

American Association of Retired Persons
1909 K Street N.W.
Washington, DC 20049
(202) 872-4700

Children of Aging Parents
2761 Trenton Road
Levittown, PA 19056
(215) 547-1070

Foundation for Hospice and Home Care
519 C Street N.E.
Washington, DC 20002
(202) 547-6586

National Council on the Aging
600 Maryland Ave. S.W.
West Wing 100
Washington, DC 20024
(202) 479-1200

National Hospice Organization
1901 North Moore Street
Suite 901
Arlington, VA 22209
(800) 658-8898

Visiting Nurse Associations of America
518 17th Street, #388
Denver CO 80202
(800) 426-2547

Sensitive and informative books are widely available. Librarians—at local community libraries and university and community libraries—and bookstore personnel are always of the utmost help in locating sources. Those titles listed here stand out as exceptionally good resources.

Recommended Reading

Callari, Elizabeth. *A Gentle Death: Personal Caregiving to the Terminally Ill.* Tudor, 1986.

Copperman, Harriet. *Dying at Home.* New York: Wiley, 1983.

Dass, Ram and Paul Gorman. *How Can I Help? Stories and Reflections on Service.* New York: Knopf, 1986.

Grollman, Earl A. *In Sickness and In Health.* Boston: Beacon, 1986.

Kaufman, Barry Neil and Suzi Lyte Kaufman. *A Land Beyond Tears: The Liberating Approach to Death and Dying.* New York: Random House, 1983 (available from Sheffield, MA: Option Indigo Press).

Kennedy, Patricia. *Dying at Home With Cancer.* Springfield: C.C. Thomas, 1982.

Kubler-Ross, Elizabeth. *Death and Dying.* New York: Macmillan, 1970.

Morra, Marion and Eve Potts. *Choices: Realistic Alternatives in Cancer Treatment.* New York: Avon, 1987.

Siegel, Bernie S., M.D. *Love, Medicine and Miracles.* New York: Harper and Row, 1988.

Strong, Maggie. *Mainstay: For the Spouse of the Chronically Ill: A Moving Personal Account and a Companion Guide.* Boston: Little, Brown, 1988.

Zimmerman, Jack. *Hospice: Complete Care for the Terminally Ill.* Boston; Urban, 1985.

INDEX

Cancer, 17, 36, 69, 70; "terminal," 35, 89-90, 95
Care, physical aspects of, 5, 97
Children, 11-12, 55-56, 64, 72, 82, 88, 98
Clergy, 4, 31, 54, 73, 94
Death, 3, 17, 20, 36, 69, 70, 88; fear of, 91-92; preparation for, 12, 40, 91-92
Denial, 35, 89-90, 94
Doctors, 47-48, 58, 73, 90, 97-99
Families, 36, 41-42, 59, 73, 74, 76, 82-83, 94-95
Grief, 24, 69, 92
Guilt, 92, 95
Helping, defined, 12-13, 97-99; kinds of, 11, 29-30, 35-43, 59, 60, 71; misconceptions, 35
Hospice, concept, 3, 17, 63, 70; definition of, 4, 37, 94; movement, 88; programs, 5, 24, 54, 70-73
Hospice team, 4-5, 23, 54, 65, 73-75, 87, 94
Hospitalization, hospice as an alternative to, 81-82, 87-95
Listening, 12, 23, 38, 42-43, 59, 98-99
Nurses, 4-5, 22-23, 39-40, 55, 65, 73, 75, 92
Pain, 5, 36, 69, 73-74, 93
Patients, emotions of, 70-71, 95; relationship to volunteer, 10, 30, 47-49, 78, 95; rights of, 58, 89-90; qualifications for hospice, 47
Primary caregivers, 29, 47, 73
Setting, 4, 70, 71-72
Social workers, 4, 65, 73, 94
Training of volunteers, 5, 9, 18, 22, 25, 53-55, 70-71, 97-99
Treatment, 36, 47-48, 90-91
Volunteers, characteristics, 17-25; disappointments, 56-58, 63-65; misconceptions, 24; limitations, 77; need for, 19, 87; personal resources, 69-78; relationships among, 55-56; rewards, 53-60, 76; screening, 24; selection, 70, 71-72; sense of humor, 23, 99; stress, 24, 69, 70, 72, 73; "typical," 21-23; qualifications, 18, 37-39; unsuitable, 24-25; value, 54, 60
Volunteer work, 24, 54-55, 56, 75-78; caseload, 78; work style, 38, 75

Dear Friend:

We would like to hear from our readers. If you have comments about this book or experiences you want to share, please write to us in care of the publisher:

Laurel Press, Inc.
1514 Holly Hill Drive
Bethel Park, PA 15102

Sally E. Lebowitz
Mary-Alice Herbert

You may order additional copies of FRIEND OF THE FAMILY direct from the publisher. For each copy, please mail $14.95 (includes postage)—Pennsylvania residents, please mail $15.85 (includes postage and 6% sales tax). Mail to: